YOUR KNOWLEDGE HAS VALUE

AF140381

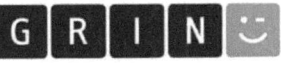

Bibliographic information published by the German National Library:

The German National Library lists this publication in the National Bibliography; detailed bibliographic data are available on the Internet at http://dnb.dnb.de .

Imprint:

Copyright © 2017 GRIN Verlag
Print and binding: Books on Demand GmbH, Norderstedt Germany
ISBN: 9783668694217

This book at GRIN:

https://www.grin.com/document/423918

Patrick Kimuyu

High Density Living as a Reliable Solution to Urban Sprawl. The Case of Sydney, Australia

GRIN Verlag

GRIN - Your knowledge has value

Since its foundation in 1998, GRIN has specialized in publishing academic texts by students, college teachers and other academics as e-book and printed book. The website www.grin.com is an ideal platform for presenting term papers, final papers, scientific essays, dissertations and specialist books.

Visit us on the internet:

http://www.grin.com/

http://www.facebook.com/grincom

http://www.twitter.com/grin_com

High Density Living Emerges as a Reliable Solution to Urban Sprawl: the Case of Sydney,

Australia

Name: Patrick Kimuyu

Content

Introduction 3

History of Housing in Sydney 3

High Density Living Internationally 4

Impact of Urban Consolidation in Sydney 7

    Urban Sprawl in Sydney 10

House VS Apartment issues Internationally 11

Apartment Development in Sydney... 12

    Melbourne, Perth and Brisbane... 14

Conclusion.. 14

References 17

Introduction

High density living is defined as 30 or more dwelling per hectare and embraces units, flats, terraces, townhouses and villas. Additionally, high density living also refers to apartment units in residential blocks of four or more storey. Majority of high density units do not have their own playing ground and share common facilities such as entrance foyers and stairwells. Urban High density living has been considered as one of the core strategies in managing urban growth (Bunker, Holloway & Randolph, 2005). In Australia, high density is considered as a vital strategy in managing the urban growth and reducing the negative impact of urban sprawl. In recent times, cities such as Sydney, Perth, Melbourne and Brisbane have been epitomized by growth in the construction of high rise apartments. Many young people prefer these kinds of dwelling since they offer advantages of location with proximity to education, jobs and other services. Various researchers points out that high density living has positive impacts such as efficient usage of land, enhanced social interaction and reduced reliance on automobiles. However, this form of living has also drawn criticism due to noise, overcrowding and limited space. The draft Metropolitan Strategy for Sydney 2031 points out that the populations will reach 1.1 million by the years 2031 hence more houses will be required (Karantonis, n.d). Therefore, this discussion paper provides a focused analysis of Sydney as a model city for high density living, a solution to urban sprawl.

History of Housing in Sydney

Sydney adopted apartment living as early as in 1930s. For example, the Australian soap opera number 96 was developed in the inner city flat which had three or more storey. According to the Gurran (2007), 20.7% of dwellings in Sydney were considered as high density in 2011. This number has increased since 1991 with more than 15.1% dwelling being drawn into this group. Notably, the highest proportion of high density flats is found in councils near the east of the CBD.

In Sydney, high density living extends by more than 20km to the west. Sydney is also experiencing a faster growth in local government areas especially those established at the centre of the middle band. Some of these LGAs include; Auburn, Parramatta (the Parramatta Road corridor) and Canada Bay. All these areas have witnessed increased growth in high density dwelling in the last twenty years (Gurran, 2007).

The current increment in the number of high density living can be attributed to the capacity offered by such housing to accommodate young families. Additionally, the changing lifestyles and structure has forced people live in high density apartments. Majority of high density apartment are located close to public amenities, restaurants, shops and employment offering attractive lifestyle to Australians (Australian Bureau of Statistics, 2004).

According to Australian Bureau of Statistics (2004 par 2), separate housing was the predominate form of housing among the Australians in 1981. Precisely, about 86% of people were living in separate dwelling. Two decades later, this number was still high with 83% of Australians sticking to separate housing. The number of Australians living in high dense apartments rose from 129,000 recorders in 1981 to about 334,000 reported in 2001.

High Density Living Internationally

According to Morris and winter (1975) theory of housing adjustment, families evaluate their housing in term of cultural and family norms. In situations where the housing does meet the norms, dissatisfaction arises, producing the prosperity of reducing the normative deficient. Modes of adjustment have to be undertaken in order to reduce the deficient. This can be achieved by residential mobility or developing mechanism for both family and residential adaptation (Samaratunga, 2013). The theory of housing adjustment is the most cited in the housing research. Ideally, the theory of housing adjustment examines housing preferences, satisfaction and the nature in which households think and performs in regard to their housing behaviors.

Charles J Stokes theory of slums can also be used to explain the socioeconomic handicaps and psychological attitudes involved in changing the socioeconomic class of low income earners living in the urban areas. According to the theory of slums, various people have divergent reasons for living in slums. Some people live in slums with the hope that their living conditions will improve. In many times, this group leaves slums to improve their economic and social standards. Majority of this group joins high density living in suburbs of big cities. The desire of living in better housing and the hopeless live of slum dwellers forces many to move to high density living (Samaratunga, 2013).

The need for housing in many cities is determined by various factors. Firstly, good shelter is seen as a vital element in assuring privacy. Many people living in slum lack privacy since they have to share essential facilities. However, with high density living, people are assured of housing that caters for all their needs. Secondly, the need for security is essential to many urban dwellers. A housing structure must offer protection, freedom from fears and stable living conditions for one's family (Samaratunga, 2013). Thirdly, many high density living comes with comfort, reputation, prestige and dignity. People prefer living in these units so as to enjoy their freedom and earn respect from their colleagues. Additionally, high dense unit comes with identity. People live in such houses in order to create a mark of identity for themselves. Ideally, an address offered by many housing units gives an individual a distinct identity. Fourthly, high dense units come with the benefit of self-expression and socializations. People live in high dense

5

units in order to relate with their friends and their neighborhood. Finally, the aesthetic nature that comes with a high dense living motivates urban dwellers in making them their homes (Samaratunga, 2013). The rising number of high rise building in the globe can also be attributed to their sustainable rent. For instance, the median weekly rent for high rise units in 2001 was ($330) while for separate houses was ($600) and that of other higher density dwellings stood at ($353). Additionally, many people prefer renting houses rather than buying hence leading to the increment of high density living in the globe (Australian Bureau of Statistics, 2004).

The increasing number of high density housing internally can be attributed to a desire to establish sustainable communities. Precisely, housing is a critical element in complex urban structures, and many city planners have a challenge in accommodating large population in small areas. Ideally, both horizontal and vertical development of the available urban land is vital in making the growing population sustainable. In order to utilize the available limited land to full capacity, a change in the housing pattern has been regarded as the best option in accommodating a greater number of people (Department of Planning, 2005).

Urban planners see high density living as the cure of avoiding the random sprawl of slums. They also argue that high density living will reduce the necessity to travel hence minimizing the energy consumption. This will lead to a reduction in pollutions since people will be living closer to their work places. Other advantages such as increased opportunities for interaction, diversity and improved access to community services will also come with high density living. Further, these buildings will also reduce the demand for public transport, car travel and the demand for parking grounds. As a result, congestion and traffic jam witnessed in many cities will reduce (Department of Planning, 2005).

The cost of building housing units is low compared to other urban houses. This is because high development of density housing can utilize scarce land in the most effective way reducing the land cost dramatically. Additionally, efficient architectural designs employed by many developers can aid in reducing the cost of infrastructural services (Samaratunga, 2013).

In Sydney and internationally, there is a perception that poor housing is a product of failed policies, inappropriate regulation, bad governance and the fundamental lack of political good will. Many governments have developed slum reduction initiatives in an effort to improve the quality of life for their people. With the aid of international bodies such as UNCHS and World Bank, improving lives of slum people is seen as the first step in making many countries economically, environmentally and culturally sustainable.

Impact of Urban Consolidation in Sydney

The first consolidation policy started in 1980 and 1981 following the government promulgation of environmental plans that supported dual occupancy. These policies gave the council the power of giving consent to development planners willing to erect two dwellings on a single block. Lack of response from these policies provoked the government to propose a state planning policy in permitting medium density housing in all residential places (Freestone, Butler-Bowdon & Randolph, 2006). The three major goals of living in high density housing included; affordability, sustainability and reducing the urban sprawl.

Precisely, the goal of urban consolidation in Sydney have been pegged at raising the number of housing units in a limited land so that they have more efficient usage of services. Additionally, the urban consolidation is aiming at reducing the overall impact on the environment while maximizing on the available land required for housing the ever increasing population. The government of Australia adopted market led consolidation by making use of the already existing residential and non-residential space and converting them into high density residential housing under ownership of private individuals. However, this process deemed unsuccessful during the initial phase since it involved unsettling of the existing residential neighborhoods majority who were poor residents (Freestone, Butler-Bowdon & Randolph, 2006). Further, these building were considered as unattractive. It was also argued that urban consolidation was the only option of reducing air pollution especially in the western Sydney which was becoming a major concern.

The government of Australia has argued that urban consolidation will reduce the cost required in infrastructural development and make full use of the existing community services. Additionally, urban consolidation will lead to low usage of fossil fuels minimizing carbon gas emissions and hence spare the environment. Evidently, the usage of fossil fuels also emits greenhouse gases which have far-reaching consequence to the environment (Searle, 2004).

High density living will also conserves both the water catchment and agricultural land since many people will be able to live in a small space. However, it should be pointed that urban consolidation can lead to spread of disease due to proximity and a high number of people. High density living have high rates of crime level hence comprising the safety of urban dwellers. Though many people are moving to high density living, some researchers argue that there has been increased traffic and overcrowding of community services (Searle, 2004). Additionally, other researchers argue that the tall building will clash the already existing neighborhood and damage the city character and image. People will be unable to move to these building to increased population leading to mental and physical illness.

Urban consolidation in Sydney can be done with various policy demands. For instance, urban consolidation leads to the establishment of a policy that encouraged energy saving and limited car use and travel. Evidently, the road transport in Australia contributes more than 88% of all emissions. The new policy will a reduce transport by automobile and help in improving the pollution problem. Additionally, more land will be left free for constructing infrastructures such as schools, hospitals and houses (Searle, 2004). The government of Australia is also planning to reduce the cost of public transport in an effort to encourage Australians make use of it. The government of Australia claimed that encouraging people to live in areas with efficient transport system such as along the bus station, and railway station will reduce the car usage and hence aid in saving fuel and energy. Ideally, train will be used to travel long distance while motor vehicles will be used to access those suburbs which cannot accommodate train. This idea has dominated zoning and development polices in both the development of high densities in outer and middle suburbs (Wright, 2006).

Urban consolidation has improved housing choice among the urban dwellers. Sydney Region Outline Plan has agitated the establishment of separate houses that could meet both single and family households with children. Providing housing in the form of townhouses, villas, units, apartments and flats provides urban dweller with many options in terms of their housing choice. It is also vital to note that urban consolidation Australia will likely decimate the urban bush land. This will affect the value of natural flora and fauna. The new plan does not allow people to have their own vegetable garden (Pears, 2005). Additionally, the housing cost will likely to soar up since land is becoming valuable in Sydney. The final cost will be passed to urban dwellers.

Notably, closer quarter living will cause problems to some people. This is because some people have been accustomed to living in single houses. Urban consolidation will make people have a high degree of tolerance since privacy will be compromised. Other problems such as noises and sharing of facilities will cause problem to city dwellers. It is vital for the government to look at the shortcomings of urban consolidation in the long run by assessing capacity of the land and infrastructure because apartments can only cater for a certain number of people. Additionally, the urban consolidation should factor the issue of children in their strategy since they have only planned single units for single families (Forster, 2006). This will avoid parents from moving to suburbs. Urban consolidation should involve all the people especially during the planning phase so as to reduce objections. Residents object urban consolidation due to doubts emanating from uncertainties such as overcrowding and environment impact of the process.

Urban Sprawl in Sydney

Population increase exerts pressure on human lives making people leave city dwelling so as to avoid unbearable life. Some people respond to the rising housing prices by relocating to the outer fringes of the city hence giving rise to urban sprawls. Majority of these fringes are poorly connected to the road system. As a result, such people tend to use motor people to access their place off work and other essential services. Additionally, fringes may turn the prime agricultural and into residential development (Bunker, Hollowayand & Randolph, 2005). According to Pears (2005), Australia is one of the most urbanized countries in the world and urban processes that have necessitated the formation of Sydney have been dynamic. In Sydney, population growth has placed pressure on health, transport, housing cost and land availability. The state government has placed in place the urban consolidation in an effort to control urban sprawl. The desire for big houses has created urban sprawls. Urban sprawls occur mostly in western Sydney concentrating within South West Growth and North West Centers. Urban sprawl has played a major role in shaping the Australian cities. However, researchers point out urban sprawl as the major source of environmental burden. This has forced the Australians government develop initiatives capable of addressing this issue. For example, the current development in Riverstone is controlled by the Australian government. The government supplements these projects with effective infrastructure, job provisions and other sustainable facilities (Bertaud & Brueckner, 2005).

Researchers argue that Sydney is one of the most expensive cities for one to live. For example, one bedroom goes for $450 to $550 a weekly while two bedroom apartments can cost a minimum of $450 to $650 on a weekly basis. Additionally, the median price to buy a house in Sydney is about $642,000 (Aura & Davidoff, 2008). However, 75% of urban dwellers prefers apartment living compared to house living.

House VS Apartment issues Internationally
House and apartment issues in Sydney and internationally have various similarities. For instance, those living in houses have the responsibility of managing all the problems affecting their surroundings. For people living in apartments, it is the responsibility of the landlord to mitigate against any issues affecting his/her tenants. It is the responsibility of the landlord to repair and maintain all the broken appliances for their tenant living in apartments. In contrast, it is the duty of a home owner to bear the full reasonability of any broken item in his/her house. Majority of apartment have bathroom, toilet and sink and landlord takes care of the plumbing activities (Bertaud & Brueckner, 2005). Further, fire control measures are also the responsibility of the landlord. Apartments have certain distinct rule that differ from those living in houses. Tenants are supposed to play low music to avoid distracting other people. Tenants are also allowed to park in spaces designated for their apartments. Further, the designated parking places

are open for competition. On the other hand, those people living in houses have the right to play their music and park in their compound. Those living in apartments have the right to modify their rooms only through the permission of the landlord. In contrast, those living in a house have the right to modify their house at their own will (Easthope & Randolph, 2009).

Houses have big space compared to apartments. For example, a small house might have 1000square feet of space while apartments have smaller than this. Some apartments cannot fit big furniture and other personal belonging and hence the need to live in a house. Living in a house for such people save money that could have been incurred in storing the items. Houses have more privacy than apartments. Living in houses relieves one the stress of adhering to stringent rules that are common in apartments (Easthope & Randolph, 2009, p. 247). Researchers' holds that the average cost of a house in Sydney is more compared to the same house in New York and London. For example, the median cost of a house in London is $462,000 compared to $651,500 in Sydney. The cost of the same house in New York is $180,000 less. This can be attributed to a high demand created by a rapid population growth.

Apartment Development in Sydney

Real estate investment is seen as a prime business both in Sydney and in the international markets. Real estate giants have made large purchases making prices for residential development houses to soar up. Additionally, the Australian government has welcomed international investors by introducing a 'Significant Investment Visa' that offers permanent residency to those companies investing a minimum of AUD$5m in a period of 4 years (Mees, 2009). The biggest beneficiary of this policy will be Chinese government which is already a force to reckon with in the real estate business. The US investment in the real estate business has doubled from in 2010-11 AUD$3.4bn to AUD$8.2bn in 2011-12. Further, UK and Singapore have also invested heavily in the real estate business. Since there is a high demand for house in Sydney, the Australian has been forced to welcome international investors. Real estate business is one of the most undertaking initiatives in the world. International developers joining Australia buy lands, design and develop the appropriate building programs. Since the development of apartment requires many skills ranging from civil engineers to surveyors, welcoming investors to Australia brings the benefits of technology transfers and employment opportunities (Mees, 2009).

Sydney like other international cities has witnessed tremendous growth in the apartment business in order to take advantage of the business niche. Evidently, real estate business and especially apartments have been developed in big cities to offer accommodation to college students and visitors attending business events, conferences and exhibitions. International investors have brought technology and capital leading to the booming business of apartments business. The Australian government aims in making Sydney the first choice global city in the Asia pacific for hosting both local and internal business. Consequently, the country will benefit economically from the apartment business (Buxton & Tieman, 2004).

Real estate business in other cities has improved communication and transportation infrastructures resulting into rapid urbanization. Australia has welcomed international investors in order to help in fighting the monopoly enjoyed by private companies. As noted earlier, Australia has witnessed urban sprawl in the last decade due to increasing prices of houses. Ideally, constructing more apartments will give the urban dwellers the variety of houses to chose from and hence improves their satisfactions. Additionally, more housing will reduce competition and reduce rent. As a result, the country will control the growth of slums (Forster, 2007).

Melbourne, Perth and Brisbane

According to Glaeser, Gyourko & Saks (2005), life is cheaper in Melbourne compared to Sydney. This implies the rent charged on Melbourne apartments is also slow. It is believed that the wealthiest class lives in Melbourne where they enjoy arts and sports. It is also argued that the unit cost of an apartment in Melbourne is $440,000. Researchers assert that Melbourne is 29% cheaper compared to Sydney. The cost of land for development is low making investors shifts their attention to Melbourne.

The cost of living in Brisbane is the cheapest compared to the other cities. The average unit price for an apartment is about $362,000. The cost of one single apartment in the city centre of Perth goes for 2,136.54 A$. This price is a bit economical since it serves mainly mine workers. It is also estimated that the average unit price for apartments in Perth stands at $411,500 (Glaeser, Gyourko & Saks, 2005). The disparities in rental prices can also be attributed to low purchasing power of inhabitants of Perth. This is because Perth is considered as an isolated town far from the capital city.

Conclusion

High density living refers to apartments blocks of four or more storey. Majority of high density apartments share common utilities. The Australian government considers high density living as a noble strategy of managing the rising population. All the three major cities in Australia have launched plans for developing high density apartments. Researchers argue that high density living enhances efficient usage of land, social interaction and reduces overreliance on automobiles. People are driven into high density apartments by a number of factors. The theory of housing adjustment holds that housing choice is determined by cultural and family norms. Additionally, the theory of slums asserts that people move from slums to high density

14

apartments in order to change their lives. High density housing is considered to offer good shelter and privacy to single families. High density housing also offers security and protection, which is lacking in slums or urban sprawls. Further, high density living come with prestige and dignity hence people is motivated to live in them. The government of Sydney considers high density living as the core strategy in attaining economic, socio-cultural and environmental sustainability.

Urban consolidation in Australia will reduce the environmental impact of fossil fuel. This is because people will be able to travel by train or live in close proximity of their working areas. Additionally, urban consolidation will conserve water and agricultural lands since the establishment of such apartments occupies a small space. Further, urban consolidation will improve housing choice and reduce cost charged from such units. Sydney like any other city is experiencing urban sprawl due to the rising population. The current housing cost charged from the apartment units are driving people to suburbs where they can afford. This will eventually raise environmental concerns in the long run.

Seemingly, various differences exist between houses and apartments. For instance, houses have high levels of privacy and the owner has the overall responsibility in managing his/her home. On the other hand, apartments are solely under landlords who have authority of their buildings. Tenants living in apartments share common facilities such as bathroom and toilet as opposed to house owners. The cost of a house in Sydney is expensive compared to the cost of the same house and apartments in international cities such as London and New York. This has led to the influx of international developers in Sydney in order to capture the already existing market. Notably, China, UK, US and Singapore have invested heavily in the real estate's business in the Australia. These investors bring innovative technology, capital and skilled labour capable of developing modern apartments and houses. The cost of a house in Melbourne is high compared to Perth and Brisbane. Brisbane is the cheapest among the cities and developers have started turning their interest in improving the town.

References

Aura, S., & Davidoff, T. (2008). Supply Constraints and Housing Prices.' *Economics Letters*, *99*(2), 275–277.

Australian Bureau of Statistics. (2004). *4102.0 - Australian Social Trends, 2004*. Retrieved from http://www.abs.gov.au/ausstats/abs@.nsf/1020492cfcd63696ca2568a1002477b5/ 939bff64e38e18ddca256e9e002912f0!OpenDocument

Bertaud, A., & Brueckner, J. (2005). Analyzing Building-Height Restrictions: Predicted Impacts and Welfare Costs. *Regional Science and Urban Economics*, *35*(2), 109–125.

Blandy, S. (2012). *Multi-owned Housing: Law, Power and Practice*. Farnham: Ashgate Publishing, Ltd.

Bunker, R., Hollowayand, D., & Randolph, B. (2005). *The social outcomes of urban consolidation in Sydney*. Retrieved from https://www.be.unsw.edu.au/sites/default/files/upload/research/centres/cf/publicat ions/researchpapers/researchpaper3.pdf

Buxton, M., & Tieman, G. (2004). *Urban Consolidation in Melbourne 1988–2003: Policy and Practice*. Melbourne: RMIT Publishing.

Department of Planning. (2005). *Metropolitan Strategy*. Sydney: City of Cities.

Easthope, H., & Randolph, B. (2009). Governing the Compact City: The Challenges of Apartment Living in Sydney, Australia. *Housing Studies*, *24*(2), 243-59.

Forster, C. (2006). The challenge of change: Australian cities and urban planning in the new millennium. *Geographical Research*, *44*(2), 173-82.

Forster, C. (2007). *Australian Cities: Continuity and Change*. South Melbourne: Oxford University Press

Freestone, R., Butler-Bowdon, C., & Randolph, W. (2006). *Talking about Sydney: Population, Community and Culture in Contemporary Sydney*. Kensington: UNSW Press.

Glaeser, L., Gyourko, J., & Saks, R. (2005). Why Have Housing Prices GoneUp? *The American Economic Review, 95*(2), 329–333.

Gurran, N. (2007). *Australian Urban Land Use Planning: Introducing Statutory Planning Practice in New South Wales*. Sydney: Sydney University Press.

Karantonis, A. (n.d). *Population growth and housing affordability in the modern city - Sydney a case study*. Retrieved from

http://www.prres.net/papers/Karantonis_Population_Growth_and_Housing_Affor dability.pdf

Mees, P. (2009). How Dense are we? Another Look at Urban Density and Transport Patterns in Australia, Canada and the USA. *Road and Transport Research, 18*(4), 58–67.

Newman, P. (2006). The environmental impact of cities. *Environment & Urbanization, 18*(2), 275-295.

Pears, A. (2005). Does Higher Density Really Reduce Household Energy Requirements? *It Depends…, Urban Policy and Research, 23*(3), 367-369.

Samaratunga, T. (2013). *LIVING SKYLINE High-Density High-Rise Low-Income Housing: An Appropriate City Planning Solution for Colombo, Sri Lanka?* Retrieved from http://epublications.bond.edu.au/cgi/viewcontent.cgi?article=1124&context=theses

Searle, G. (2004). The limits to urban consolidation. *Australian Planner, 41*(1), 42-48.

Wright, K. (2006). The Relationship between Residential Density and Non-Transport Energy Use. *Australian Planner, 43*(4), 12-13.

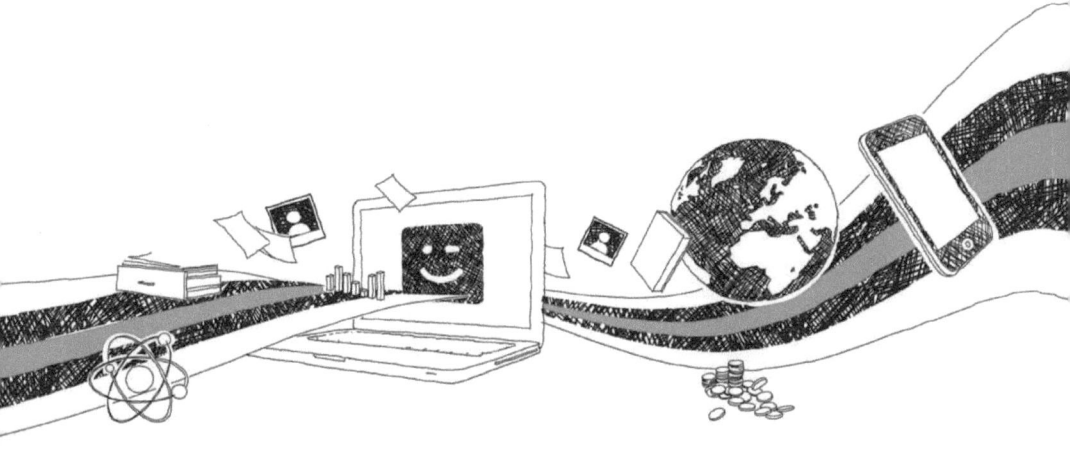
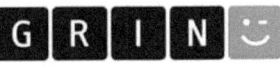